The powerful ways of controlling high and low blood pressure

Sandra J. Hill

Table of Contents

FOREWORD

Pulse is a principal part of cardiovascular wellbeing that alludes to the power applied by flowing blood against the walls of the conduits. Understanding circulatory strain is fundamental since it assists with forestalling and oversees different medical conditions, like coronary illness, stroke, and kidney harm. Two numbers are used to measure blood pressure: systolic pressure, which is the pressure when the heart contracts, and diastolic pressure, which is the pressure when the heart rests between beats. Maintaining healthy blood pressure levels is essential to avoiding the risk of developing serious health issues, and it is an essential part of regular health checkups.

CHAPTER1

What is Hypertension

Hypertension, otherwise called hypertension, is a typical condition that happens when the circulatory strain in the supply routes is constantly raised. Hypertension is a serious medical condition that can prompt coronary illness, stroke, and different intricacies. Hypertension is a silent killer because its symptoms rarely surface. On the other hand, some individuals may experience nosebleeds, shortness of breath, or headaches. Natural methods for lowering blood pressure include incorporating stress management, regular exercise, and a well-balanced diet. High blood pressure can sometimes be controlled with medication.

A condition known as hypotension or low blood pressure is one in which the blood pressure in the arteries is lower than normal. Low blood pressure can make you feel dizzy, faint, and tired. Dehydration, heart issues, and certain medications are all possible causes. Low blood pressure can be managed with lifestyle changes like drinking more fluids, eating smaller, frequent meals, and not getting up too quickly. In most cases, low blood pressure is not a serious health issue. However, if low blood pressure is severe and does not go away, it may necessitate medical intervention or medication.

In conclusion, maintaining overall health and avoiding serious health issues require an understanding of blood pressure. Circulatory strain is a crucial sign that mirrors the power of blood against the walls of the conduits. Common conditions like hypotension and hypertension require care and attention. Managing blood pressure and lowering the risk of complications can be accomplished through lifestyle changes and medication. Standard pulse checks, solid way of life propensities, and clinical mediation when fundamental can assist people with keeping up with sound circulatory strain levels. Circulatory strain is a fundamental proportion of the power that your heart uses to siphon blood all through your body. Pulse is estimated by two numbers, the systolic and diastolic tensions, and is communicated in millimeters of mercury (mmHg).

CHAPTER2

Systolic and diastolic are the two numbers used to measure blood pressure, The highest number in the reading is the systolic pressure, which measures the force of blood against your arteries when your heart beats. The diastolic tension is the base number in the perusing, and it estimates the power of blood against the walls of your veins when your heart is very still between thumps. Pulse is a significant mark of generally wellbeing, and it can assist with diagnosing conditions like hypertension.

A sphygmomanometer, made up of a pressure gauge and an inflatable cuff, is typically used to take blood pressure readings. The brachial artery is compressed by inflating the cuff, which is wrapped around the upper arm. The pressure inside the cuff is then measured by the pressure gauge, which is the force of blood against the artery walls. The ratio of systolic pressure to diastolic pressure is how blood pressure is measured. A systolic pressure of 120 mmHg and a diastolic pressure of 80 mmHg, for instance, would be indicated by a reading of 120/80 mmHg.

Pulse is a significant mark of generally speaking wellbeing, and it can assist with diagnosing conditions like hypertension. Hypertension is a condition wherein the power of blood against the walls of your courses is reliably excessively high. This can prompt an assortment of medical conditions, including coronary illness, stroke, and kidney infection. Regular blood pressure checks are essential because hypertension often goes unnoticed. If you have high blood pressure, your doctor may advise you to make changes to your lifestyle, like exercising and changing your diet, or to take medication to lower your blood pressure.

In conclusion, blood pressure is an important indicator of how much force your heart uses to move blood around your body. The systolic and diastolic pressures, which are the two numbers used to measure blood pressure, are expressed in millimeters of mercury (mmHg). A sphygmomanometer, made up of a pressure gauge and an inflatable cuff, is typically used to take blood pressure readings. Blood pressure is an essential measure of the health of the cardiovascular system, and it can assist in the diagnosis of conditions such as hypertension. Blood pressure is an important indicator of overall health. It is the force that the blood exerts as it moves through the body against the walls of the blood vessels. Pulse is estimated in millimeters of mercury (mmHg), and it is communicated as two numbers: systolic tension (the larger number) and diastolic strain (the lower number). It is possible to measure blood pressure at home or in a doctor's office using a straightforward and non-invasive procedure.

Using a sphygmomanometer, which consists of a stethoscope, a pressure gauge, and an inflatable cuff, is the most common way to measure blood pressure. The pressure gauge is used to inflate the cuff until the blood flow stops. The cuff is wrapped around the upper arm. After that, the stethoscope is used to listen to the sounds of blood flowing through the brachial artery as the pressure is gradually released. The principal sound heard is the systolic tension, and the last strong heard is the diastolic strain.

Individuals who wish to take their own blood pressure readings can also purchase home blood pressure monitors. There are two kinds of these easy-to-use devices: automatic and manual The user of a manual blood pressure monitor must use a stethoscope to listen for the sounds of blood flow and inflate the cuff. Because they are simple to operate and do not require any special skills, automatic monitors are becoming increasingly popular. They come with a cuff that automatically inflates, and a digital screen shows the readings.

In conclusion, maintaining good cardiovascular health necessitates an understanding of blood pressure. It is possible to measure blood pressure at home or in a doctor's office using a straightforward and non-invasive procedure. A sphygmomanometer is the most common instrument used to measure blood pressure, but home blood pressure monitors are also available for those who prefer to monitor their own blood pressure on their own. It is recommended to measure blood pressure at various times to obtain an accurate picture of one's blood pressure because it is important to keep in mind that blood pressure readings can fluctuate throughout the day.

One of the most vital signs in the human body is blood pressure. It is the power of the blood pushing against the walls of the veins as the heart siphons. A pulse perusing comprises of two numbers, systolic and diastolic. The unit of measurement for these values is millimeters of mercury (mmHg). Pulse readings are communicated as systolic over diastolic, like 120/80 mmHg.

Deciphering circulatory strain numbers is pivotal to grasping the gamble of creating cardiovascular infections. The systolic number addresses the strain in the courses when the heart beats or agreements. The pressure in the arteries when the heart is at rest in between beats is represented by the diastolic number. When the systolic number is less than 120 mmHg and the diastolic number is less than 80 mmHg, blood pressure is considered normal. Hypertension, otherwise called hypertension, is analyzed when the systolic number is 130 mmHg or higher, or the diastolic number is 80 mmHg or higher. A high risk of developing high blood pressure is indicated by a blood pressure reading between 120/80 mmHg and 129/80 mmHg.

It is essential to comprehend that various factors, including stress, physical activity, and medication, can cause blood pressure readings to fluctuate throughout the day. In order to obtain an accurate reading, multiple readings at various times are suggested. Heart attack, stroke, and kidney disease are just a few of the serious health issues that can result from high blood pressure. Maintaining a healthy lifestyle, which includes regular exercise, eating a well-balanced diet, and avoiding smoking and excessive alcohol consumption, is essential for controlling blood pressure. High blood pressure can sometimes be controlled with medication. In general, maintaining good cardiovascular health requires an understanding of blood pressure numbers.

The force at which blood moves through your veins and arteries is known as blood pressure. It is communicated in two numbers — the systolic strain (top number) and the diastolic tension (base number). The ordinary pulse is around 120/80 mmHg. However, high blood pressure can result in serious health issues such as kidney damage, heart disease, and stroke. In this manner, it is fundamental to oversee circulatory strain levels to keep up with ideal wellbeing. Although it can be difficult, controlling blood pressure is not impossible.

CHAPTER3

The Methods for controlling blood pressure.

Here are some efficient methods for controlling blood pressure. The most important thing is to keep a healthy weight. Being overweight or corpulent can essentially expand the gamble of hypertension. To maintain a healthy weight, one should eat a well-balanced diet and exercise frequently. Additionally, lowering blood pressure levels can be aided by decreasing sodium intake and increasing potassium intake. Finally, reducing alcohol intake and quitting smoking can both aid in blood pressure control.

However, constant effort and monitoring are necessary for blood pressure management. It is essential to monitor blood pressure levels on a regular basis to identify any changes and take the necessary actions. Using a blood pressure monitor, one can check their own blood pressure at home or by visiting a doctor. It is additionally fundamental to adhere to prescription guidelines endorsed by the medical care supplier. Skipping prescription dosages or halting medicine unexpectedly can prompt abrupt spikes in pulse levels. As a result, one should adhere to the medication schedule and talk to their doctor about any concerns or side effects.

All in all, overseeing circulatory strain levels is critical for keeping up with ideal wellbeing. Some effective strategies for controlling blood pressure include reducing alcohol consumption, quitting smoking, eating a well-balanced diet, engaging in regular physical activity, consuming less sodium, quitting smoking, and maintaining a healthy weight. Also, customary checking of circulatory strain levels and adhering to medicine guidelines endorsed by the medical services supplier are fundamental. One can effectively control their blood pressure and lower their risk of serious health problems by following these steps.

Hypertension, otherwise called hypertension, is a condition where the power of blood against the walls of the veins is reliably high. Whenever left unmanaged, it can prompt serious medical conditions like coronary illness, stroke, and kidney disappointment. Fortunately, there are a number of options for controlling high blood pressure and minimizing the likelihood of complications.

Changing one's lifestyle is the first step in controlling high blood pressure. This incorporates keeping a sound weight, eating a reasonable eating routine low in sodium and high in products of the soil, getting ordinary actual work, stopping smoking, and restricting liquor consumption. Rolling out these improvements can assist with bringing down circulatory strain and work on in general wellbeing.

High blood pressure may require medication in addition to

lifestyle adjustments. Diuretics, ACE inhibitors, beta-blockers, and calcium channel blockers are some of the classes of drugs that can be used. It means quite a bit to work with a medical services supplier to decide the best drug routine in view of individual necessities and inclinations. In order to guarantee that treatment is working and that any necessary adjustments can be made, regular blood pressure monitoring is also essential. Generally, overseeing hypertension requires a blend of way of life changes and prescription to diminish the gamble of intricacies and work on by and large wellbeing.

Hypertension, otherwise called hypertension, is a typical condition that influences a huge number of individuals around the world. It is portrayed by the power of blood against the walls of your supply routes being excessively high, which can prompt serious medical conditions like coronary illness, stroke, and kidney harm. Luckily, there are numerous ways of overseeing hypertension, including way of life changes and drugs. In this article, we will zero in on meds that are usually used to oversee hypertension.

High blood pressure can be controlled with a variety of medications, each of which lowers blood pressure in a different way. The absolute most normal drugs incorporate diuretics, ACE inhibitors, calcium channel blockers, and beta-blockers. Diuretics work by eliminating abundance water and salt from your body, which assists with diminishing the volume of blood in your corridors and lower your circulatory strain. Expert inhibitors work by hindering the development of a chemical called angiotensin II, which makes your veins slender and your pulse to increment. Calcium channel blockers work by loosening up the muscles in your veins, which permits them to enlarge and works on the progression of blood. In addition to lowering your blood pressure, beta-blockers work by reducing the force of your heartbeat and slowing your heart rate.

It is vital to take note of that drugs ought to constantly be taken as coordinated by your PCP, and you ought to take constantly them without speaking with your medical care supplier. This is due to the fact that high blood pressure frequently goes unnoticed, and if you stop taking your medication, it could cause your blood pressure to rise to dangerous levels without your knowledge. Also, it might require an investment to find the right medicine or mix of prescriptions that turns out best for you, so it is vital to be patient and work intimately with your primary care physician to find the right treatment plan. It is possible to manage high blood pressure and lower your risk of serious health issues with the right medications and lifestyle changes.

Hypertension, also known as high blood pressure, is a common condition that affects millions of people worldwide. Because it can cause serious health issues like heart disease, stroke, and kidney failure without causing any obvious symptoms, it is often referred to as the "silent killer." Changing one's lifestyle is an important part of controlling high blood pressure, which is necessary to avoid these problems.

Changing one's lifestyle in a way that lowers blood pressure is one of the best ways to control high blood pressure. These progressions incorporate keeping a sound weight, participating in ordinary actual work, decreasing salt admission, and restricting liquor utilization. Getting thinner can assist with bringing down circulatory strain levels, and it can likewise decrease the gamble of creating other medical conditions, like diabetes and coronary illness. Standard activity, like strolling, swimming, or cycling, can assist with bringing down pulse levels and work on generally cardiovascular wellbeing.

In general, controlling high blood pressure requires monitoring and maintaining healthy levels. Keeping track of blood pressure levels can be made easier with home blood pressure monitors and regular visits to the doctor. A healthy diet and regular exercise, in addition to any medication that may be prescribed, can assist in maintaining healthy blood pressure levels and preventing serious health issues. People can effectively manage their high blood pressure and improve their overall health and well-being by taking these steps.

CHAPTER4

How to manage high blood pressure,

For managing high blood pressure, it's also important to cut back on salt intake. Salt can lead to water retention in the body, which can raise blood pressure. Restricting salt admission by keeping away from handled food varieties and planning feasts at home can assist with decreasing circulatory strain levels. At long last, restricting liquor utilization can likewise assist with bringing down pulse levels, as liquor can increment circulatory strain and add to other medical conditions, like liver sickness and malignant growth.

Taking everything into account, overseeing hypertension is fundamental for forestalling serious medical conditions, and way of life changes are a significant piece of this interaction. Keeping a healthy weight, getting regular exercise, cutting back on salt and alcohol, and drinking less are all good ways to lower blood pressure and improve overall health. By making these way of life changes, individuals with hypertension can diminish their gamble of creating inconveniences and work on their personal satisfaction.

Seeing a doctor on a regular basis is essential for keeping track of blood pressure levels. Using a stethoscope, an inflatable cuff, a pressure gauge, and a sphygmomanometer, they can measure your blood pressure. Additionally, there are home blood pressure monitors that can be purchased and utilized for daily monitoring of blood pressure. It is vital to adhere to the guidelines for use cautiously and to have the gadget aligned routinely.

Keeping up with sound pulse levels can be accomplished through way of life changes and medicine, whenever endorsed by a medical care supplier. Maintaining a healthy weight, eating a balanced diet high in fruits and vegetables and low in sodium, exercising regularly, limiting alcohol intake, and quitting smoking are all examples of lifestyle changes. Blood pressure can also be reduced with medication like diuretics, ACE inhibitors, and calcium channel blockers. It's important to talk to a doctor about your options for treatment and to follow their advice for controlling high blood pressure.

Circulatory strain is the proportion of the power of blood against the walls of the conduits as it courses through the body. Hypertension, otherwise called hypertension, is a condition where the pulse in the corridors is reliably raised over the typical reach. A condition in which the blood pressure in the arteries consistently falls below the normal range is known as hypotension. There are natural treatments for managing high and low blood pressure, both of which can result in serious health issues.

CHAPTER5

What are the treatments for high blood pressure?

Natural treatments for high blood pressure include eating a healthy diet high in potassium and low in sodium. This implies consuming a lot of natural products, vegetables, entire grains, and lean proteins. Furthermore, normal activity, keeping a sound weight, and lessening pressure can likewise assist with bringing down pulse. It has also been demonstrated that some supplements and herbs, like fish oil, garlic, and hibiscus, can lower blood pressure.

For low pulse, regular cures incorporate expanding liquid and salt admission, which can assist with raising circulatory strain. It is also possible to maintain stable blood pressure by eating small, frequent meals throughout the day. Furthermore, abstaining from representing delayed timeframes, wearing pressure stockings, and gradually ascending from a situated or lying position can likewise assist with forestalling an unexpected drop in circulatory strain. It has also been demonstrated that some supplements and herbs, like ginseng and licorice root, can raise blood pressure.

It is essential to keep in mind that medical treatment for high or low blood pressure should not be used in place of natural remedies. It means a lot to work with a medical services supplier to screen pulse and decide the best course of therapy. Natural remedies, on the other hand, can be an effective way to control blood pressure and improve overall health in a treatment plan.

Practice is a characteristic solution for both high and low

pulse. Ordinary activity can assist lower with high blooding strain by fortifying the heart, further developing blood stream, and decreasing how much work the heart needs to do to siphon blood all through the body. Exercise can likewise assist raise with low blooding strain by further developing course and expanding blood volume.

For those with hypertension, it is prescribed to participate in vigorous activity for somewhere around 30 minutes out of every day most days of the week. This can incorporate exercises like energetic strolling, cycling, swimming, or moving. Additionally, resistance training can help lower blood pressure. It is vital to begin gradually and bit by bit increment the force and span of activity to keep away from injury.

For those with low circulatory strain, exercise can be useful in raising pulse. Prescribed to participate in exercises increment pulse and animate course, like strolling, running, or cycling. To ensure safety, it is essential to keep hydrated, avoid overheating, and monitor blood pressure before, during, and after exercise.

In conclusion, both high and low blood pressure can be naturally treated with exercise. By improving circulation, strengthening the heart, and reducing the amount of work the heart must do, regular exercise can assist in lowering high blood pressure and raising low blood pressure. In order to stay safe, it's important to start slowly and gradually increase the intensity and duration of exercise. Additionally, it's important to keep an eye on your blood pressure before, during, and after exercise. It can be simple and effective to manage blood pressure and

improve overall health to
incorporate exercise into daily
routine.

CHAPTER6

Natural remedies for controlling high blood pressure,

Many people around the world suffer from high blood pressure, which is a prevalent condition. Natural remedies can also be effective in controlling high blood pressure, despite the fact that some medications can treat it. Techniques for reducing stress are one of the natural remedies for high blood pressure that works best. Stress can make the veins tighten, prompting hypertension. By diminishing pressure, you can bring down your circulatory strain and work on your general wellbeing.

There are many pressure decrease strategies that you can use to control your circulatory strain. One of the best strategies is profound relaxing. Deep breathing aids in stress reduction and body relaxation. Sitting comfortably and taking slow, deep breaths is a good way to practice deep breathing. Meditation is yet another effective method for dealing with stress. Meditation aids in stress reduction and mental clarity. Sitting in a quiet place and concentrating on your breath or a mantra is one way to engage in meditation.

You can control your blood pressure with the help of other stress-relieving strategies, such as deep breathing and meditation. These incorporate yoga, jujitsu, and moderate muscle unwinding. Yoga and tai chi are ancient practices that combine meditation, physical postures, and breathing exercises to alleviate stress and improve health in general. In order to alleviate stress and encourage relaxation, progressive muscle relaxation involves contracting and relaxing various muscle groups. By integrating these pressure decrease methods into your everyday daily schedule, you have some control over your pulse and work on your general wellbeing.

Many people around the world suffer from high blood pressure, which is a prevalent condition. Natural remedies can also be effective in controlling high blood pressure, despite the fact that some medications can treat it. Techniques for reducing stress are one of the natural remedies for high blood pressure that works best. Stress can make the veins choke, prompting hypertension. You can lower your blood pressure and improve your overall health by reducing stress.

There are many pressure decrease methods that you can use to control your pulse. Deep breathing is one of the most effective techniques. Deep breathing aids in stress reduction and body relaxation. You can rehearse profound breathing by sitting in an agreeable position and taking sluggish, full breaths. Another viable pressure decrease method is contemplation. Contemplation assists with quieting the psyche and lessen pressure. Sitting in a quiet place and concentrating on your breath or a mantra is one way to engage in meditation.

As well as profound breathing and contemplation, there are other pressure decrease methods that you can use to control your circulatory strain. Yoga, tai chi, and progressive muscle relaxation are a few examples. Yoga and jujitsu are old practices that join actual stances, breathing methods, and contemplation to decrease pressure and work on by and large wellbeing. In order to alleviate stress and encourage relaxation, progressive muscle relaxation involves contracting and relaxing various muscle groups. You can control your blood pressure and improve your overall health by incorporating these stress-reduction strategies into your daily routine.

CHAPTER 7
Dietary changes

Normal cures can be a protected and compelling method for overseeing high and low circulatory strain. One of the main ways of controlling pulse is through dietary changes. Hypertension, otherwise called hypertension, can frequently be overseen by diminishing how much salt and immersed fat in the eating regimen. Low circulatory strain, otherwise called hypotension, can be overseen by expanding the admission of liquids, salt, and caffeine.

It is essential to eat less sodium in order to control high blood pressure. Because a lot of packaged and processed foods contain sodium, it is important to read food labels and choose foods with less sodium. Saturated fat consumption reduction can also help control blood pressure. This can be accomplished by avoiding red meat and full-fat dairy products and choosing lean protein sources like fish, chicken breast, and legumes.

To oversee low pulse, it is vital to build the admission of liquids, salt, and caffeine. It is possible to maintain blood pressure and increase blood volume by drinking a lot of water and other fluids. Also, expanding the admission of salt can assist with raising pulse, however it is vital to do as such with some restraint. Before making any significant dietary changes, it is essential to consult a healthcare professional because excessive salt consumption can have adverse effects on one's health. Caffeine can also lower blood pressure, but it should be taken in moderation and not in excessive quantities.

In general, dietary changes can be a powerful method for overseeing both high and low pulse. By lessening the admission of sodium and immersed fat and expanding the admission of liquids, salt, and caffeine depending on the situation, people can direct their pulse normally and securely. Nonetheless, it is vital to talk with a medical care supplier prior to rolling out any huge improvements to the eating regimen, as need might arise and ailments can shift.

A medical condition known as hypotension or low blood pressure occurs when the blood pressure in the arteries falls below the normal range. This condition can result in fainting, dizziness, and, in severe cases, shock. It is essential to prevent low blood pressure, particularly for those who have a history of it or are at risk of developing it.

One of the best ways of forestalling low pulse is by remaining hydrated. A drop in blood pressure, which can result in fainting and dizziness, can be caused by dehydration. To keep the body's electrolytes in the right balance, it's critical to drink enough water and other fluids. Moreover, eating food varieties that are wealthy in sodium can assist with keeping up with circulatory strain levels. However, before increasing their sodium intake, individuals with high blood pressure should consult their physicians.

One more method for forestalling low circulatory strain is by keeping away from unexpected changes in pose. Standing up excessively fast or sitting for expanded periods can cause an unexpected drop in pulse. People should take their time when changing positions and avoid sitting or standing for too long to avoid this. By improving blood circulation and maintaining a healthy weight, regular exercise can also aid in the prevention of low blood pressure.

In conclusion, it is essential to prevent low blood pressure because it can be a serious medical condition. Several ways to prevent this condition include drinking enough water, eating enough sodium, and avoiding sudden posture changes. People who are in danger of growing low circulatory strain ought to counsel their PCPs for customized exhortation on the best way to forestall this condition. Individuals can avoid complications associated with low blood pressure and maintain healthy blood pressure levels by following these straightforward steps.

A medical condition known as hypotension or low blood pressure occurs when blood pressure falls below the normal range. This can result in organ damage, fainting, and dizziness in severe cases. While some people have low blood pressure by nature, others may be affected by certain medications or health conditions. Fortunately, there are a number of ways to avoid having low blood pressure.

First and foremost, remaining hydrated is a compelling method for forestalling low circulatory strain. A drop in blood volume, which can result in a decrease in blood pressure, can be caused by dehydration. It is prescribed to drink somewhere around eight glasses of water each day to guarantee appropriate hydration. Furthermore, keeping away from liquor and caffeine can likewise assist with forestalling low pulse, as these substances can make parchedness and lead a drop in circulatory strain.

Besides, keeping a sound eating regimen can likewise help

with forestalling low pulse. Salty foods can raise blood pressure, which helps prevent hypotension. Nonetheless, it is essential to take note of that people with specific ailments, like coronary illness, ought to restrict their salt admission. Also, consuming little, successive dinners over the course of the day can assist with forestalling drops in glucose, which can prompt low pulse.

Lastly, regular exercise can also assist in the prevention of low blood pressure. Exercise improves blood flow and strengthens the heart, both of which can keep blood pressure from dropping.

However, in order to prevent drops in blood pressure during and after physical activity, it is essential to begin slowly and gradually increase the intensity and duration of exercise. People with specific medical issue ought to talk with their medical services supplier prior to beginning a work-out daily practice to guarantee security.

In conclusion, there are a number of ways to prevent low blood pressure, such as staying hydrated, eating a healthy diet, and exercising frequently. People can avoid the negative effects of low blood pressure and maintain their overall health and wellbeing by implementing these strategies. If you start a new exercise or diet regimen or if you have symptoms of low blood pressure, it is important to talk to a doctor.

A condition in which the blood pressure falls below normal levels is referred to as low blood pressure or hypotension. Although low blood pressure may not always be a cause for concern, if it is severe or causes symptoms like fainting or dizziness, it can be dangerous.

CHAPTER 8

What are the reasons for low pulse?

There are a few reasons for low pulse, and it is essential to comprehend them to forestall the condition and oversee it really.

One of the most widely recognized reasons for low pulse is parchedness. At the point when the body loses a larger number of liquids than it takes in, it can prompt a drop in pulse. Different causes incorporate specific meds, like diuretics and beta-blockers, as well as heart issues, endocrine problems, and nerve harm. Low blood pressure can occur as a side effect of pregnancy or as a result of rising too quickly from a seated or prone position.

The side effects of low pulse can shift contingent upon the reason and seriousness of the condition. Normal side effects incorporate discombobulating, tipsiness, swooning, obscured vision, queasiness, and exhaustion. Now and again, low circulatory strain may likewise cause windedness, chest agony, or disarray. On the off chance that you experience any of these side effects, it is vital to look for clinical consideration immediately, as they might show a more serious basic condition.

To forestall low pulse, it is essential to remain hydrated, particularly during blistering climate or while participating in actual work. Talk to your doctor about adjusting your dosage or switching to a different medication if you are currently taking any medications that have the potential to lower your blood pressure. When standing up, if you tend to have low blood pressure, try to do so slowly and avoid making sudden movements. Low blood pressure can be effectively controlled and monitored with proper prevention and treatment.

If not properly managed, hypotension, or low blood pressure, can result in a variety of issues. It can cause tipsiness, swooning, exhaustion, and even organ harm in extreme cases. Accordingly, it is pivotal to do whatever it takes to forestall low circulatory strain. The importance of staying hydrated is one of the most important things to keep in mind.

Our blood volume decreases when we are dehydrated, causing our blood pressure to drop. This can be particularly dangerous for individuals who as of now have low pulse. In this way, drinking a lot of liquids over the course of the day is fundamental. Water is the most ideal choice, yet different refreshments like tea and organic product juice can likewise add to your liquid admission. It's important to remember that drinking alcohol and caffeine can actually make you dehydrated, so it's best to limit how much you drink.

Consuming foods that are high in water content is another way to keep hydrated. Leafy foods like watermelon, cucumber, and celery are extraordinary decisions. Because they contain both water and electrolytes, broths and soups are also excellent choices. Electrolytes are minerals like sodium, potassium, and magnesium that assistance to manage liquid equilibrium in the body. Electrolytes are lost when we sweat or urinate, so it's important to eat to get them back.

In conclusion, one of the most crucial steps you can take to prevent low blood pressure is to drink enough water. By drinking a lot of liquids and eating water-rich food sources, you can assist with keeping up with your blood volume and forestall drops in circulatory strain. In the event that you are inclined to low circulatory strain, it's particularly essential to remain hydrated and stay away from drying out however much as could reasonably be expected. Keep in mind, anticipation is key with regards to overseeing low pulse, so make a point to focus on your hydration needs.

If not treated properly, low blood pressure is a medical condition that can cause dizziness, fainting, and even shock. One of the primary drivers of low pulse is the utilization of specific prescriptions. Avoiding these medications is essential for those who are at risk of developing low blood pressure.

Low blood pressure can be brought on by a variety of drugs. These include medications for high blood pressure, diuretics, antidepressants, and Parkinson's disease treatments. The blood vessels may dilate as a result of these medications, lowering blood pressure. Patients taking these medications should keep an eye on their blood pressure on a regular basis and inform their doctor of any significant changes.

It is essential to discuss any medication changes with a healthcare provider in order to avoid low blood pressure. People who are in danger of growing low circulatory strain ought to likewise keep away from liquor and caffeine, as these substances can likewise make veins widen and prompt a drop in pulse. Maintaining healthy blood pressure levels can also be helped by drinking enough water and eating well.

In general, controlling high blood pressure is an important part of staying healthy. People can lower their risk of developing low blood pressure by avoiding medications that can cause it. It is critical to examine any drug changes with a medical care supplier and to screen circulatory strain consistently to guarantee that it stays inside a solid reach. People can maintain their health and avoid the negative effects of low blood pressure by following these steps.

THE END

www.ingramcontent.com/pod-product-compliance
Lightning Source LLC
Chambersburg PA
CBHW070037260726

48658CB00002B/657